HEALTHY SKIN;

Cook. Nourish. Glow. 50 Beginner Snacks, Meals and Smoothies For Glowing Skin, Skin Cleanser

By

Angela Knightsbridge

Table of Contents

Introduction

I want to thank you for purchasing 'Healthy Skin; Cook. Nourish. Glow. 50 Beginner Snacks, Meals and Smoothies for Glowing Skin.'

Let me start by saying this book contains proven research into nutrition that will not only greatly improve your skin and general health, but are also easy to prepare and mouth-wateringly delicious.

We all have our favourite face cream or treatment, but beautiful skin starts from within. A steady supply of the right micronutrients is essential to supporting the shedding of older skin cells which are replaced by new ones - thus giving us a youthful look!

I have coached numerous clients to get fit and healthy from the inside out using these exact recipes. I firmly believe that you can eat a healthy diet to look your very best without expensive creams. Everybody can cook delicious, healthy, beautiful food to look gorgeous.

A fact about your skin: Everyday it is under a constant attack from a barrage of daily pollutants and bad diet choices all designed to age, blemish and make us look wrinkled.

- Smoking, pollution and too much sunlight can cause wrinkling and age spots.
- Repeatedly losing and regaining weight can take its toll on your skin and can cause sagging and wrinkles.
- Severe crash diets are often short of essential vitamins and minerals too and can have a damaging effect on your skin.
- Lack of hydration can cause your skin to look dry and wrinkled.

However, all is not lost. We have the answer; if we eat the correct balance of foods, you'll feed your skin the vital nutrients it needs to help it stay soft, supple and blemish-free. Fruit and vegetables are top of the list and contain powerful antioxidants that help to protect skin from the cellular damage caused by free radicals.

With this book we will develop your instincts for choosing quick snacks, to make easy meals, all jam-packed full of nutrients. As an example Beta-carotene, found in pumpkin, carrots and sweet potatoes, and lutein, found in kale, papaya and spinach among others are full of potent antioxidants, which is vital for normal skin cell development.

It's time for you to become an expert at not only regenerating your skin to its former glory, but to have the best skin you ever had, glowing, healthy and radiant. Let's begin this journey.

Chapter 1: Breakfasts

The thing about the foods you will find in this chapter and others, is that you most likely already eat them. You might not eat them often or you might be eating them every meal. When you eat a well-balanced breakfast, with vegetables, fruit, eggs, oatmeal, and other suggestions found in here, you are getting the antioxidants, anti-inflammatories, and collagen your skin needs to remain healthy. A combination of vitamin C, D, E, A, K, and beta-carotene found in pumpkin, carrots, and other orange fruits all provide collagen and properties to rejuvenate your skin.

1. Green Eggs and Ham Omelet

Are you a fan of green eggs and ham? Well, we have a new take on the children's favorite that you can incorporate into a delicious, fun and nutrition packed breakfast. The secret to this delightful addition is spinach. The fact is, spinach is one of the best ways to keep you healthy and glowing.

Ingredients:

- 2 eggs
- 1 slice of ham or half cup cubed
- 1 ounce or 1 slice of cheddar cheese
- ½ cup fresh small leaf spinach
- ¼ cup chopped green pepper

Combine all the ingredients into your nutrition blender to mix until blended. The pan should be preheated and sprayed with cooking oil or butter. Cook until done. Serves one.

2. Fruit Salad with Tropical Feel

Antioxidants abound in this "feel the ocean breeze" fruit salad. Not only will your skin reap the benefits of the fresh fruit ingredients, the potassium from cantaloupe and bananas are good for keeping your blood pressure lower. Potassium is also a known ingredient to prevent cramps in your limbs.

Ingredients:

- 1 cup vanilla yogurt, low fat

- 1 teaspoon grated lime zest

- 2 red grapefruits

- 2 kiwi fruit, peeled and cut into small wedges

- 2 bananas, sliced

- 1 small cantaloupe, cut into chunks

- 1 large papaya, seeded and cut into chunks

- 2 tablespoons crystallized ginger

Combine first two ingredients in a small bowl. Prepare the fruits in a large bowl, sectioning the grapefruits over the bowl to catch the juices Squeeze the peels to get all the juice from the membranes. Add the rest of the fruit and ginger. This serves six. Divide the fruit into small bowls and top with the yogurt mixture.

3. Frittata with Zucchini

Zucchini is a rich source of flavonoids, that harm free radicals, which play a role in the aging process. It is low in calories and contain a wonderful bounty of vitamin C another good antioxidant. Add juice or fresh fruit and you have another skin protector against aging.

Ingredients:

- 4 eggs
- 4 egg whites
- ¼ cup of Parmesan cheese
- ¼ teaspoon Mediterranean Sea salt
- 2 tablespoons olive oil
- 1 clove, minced garlic
- 2 small zucchinis, shredded
- 2 red peppers, cut into strips

Eggs provide the protein and using half the yolks ensure that cholesterol levels are kept in check. Preheat the oven to 400 degrees. In a medium bowl, whisk the first four ingredients. Heat oil in a skillet that can be placed in the oven, add garlic and cook for one minute or until just tender. Add the zucchini and peppers and cook for another minute. Pour in the egg mixture and cook about three minutes or until the bottom of the mixture is set. Bake in the oven to finish cooking, about ten minutes.

4. Oatmeal with Berries and Spice

Oatmeal is another staple to have on your pantry shelf. Adding berries, spices, and nuts to the bowl, will add the antioxidants you need for a glowing complexion. The nutrients in this power food support skin health. Add a hardboiled egg for protein and you have a great way to begin your day.

Ingredients:

- ½ cup oatmeal, steel cut, rolled or quick cooking

- ¼ cup berries, blueberries, strawberries, peaches, raspberries, or bananas

- 1/8 teaspoon pumpkin spice

- 1/8 cup chopped nuts, walnuts, pecans, or almonds

Prepare oatmeal according to package directions. If you use steel cut oatmeal you can make a family breakfast in a slow cooker. Wake up to a delicious meal without the fuss. Use 1 cup of oats to 3 cups of water. After the oatmeal is cooked, add the spice, berries and nuts. A sprinkle of brown sugar can be added to taste.

5. Breakfast Sandwich with Kale

If you like a breakfast sandwich you can find a great one for your skin with kale. Don't think traditional breakfast muffin, these delightful gems are cooked in a muffin tin with eggs.

Ingredients:

- Kale
- Half dozen eggs
- Peppers
- Onions
- Mushrooms
- Milk or Coconut Milk

Combine the ingredients into a blender, mix into a smooth consistency, add a tsp milk or coconut milk per egg, whip, and put in a muffin tin. Bake at 350 degrees F for 10 to 15 minutes, or until egg is fully cooked. You can also substitute for other vegetables. Any vegetables mentioned in this chapter that are good for skin glow can be used in your egg muffin.

6. Italian Omelet

The Italian omelet is going to provide eggs, which are healthy for your heart. It also contains tomatoes, which are known to help fight sunburn, reduce skin roughness, and boost collagen.

Ingredients:

- 1 Tbsp. chopped green bell pepper

- 1 Tbsp. chopped onion

- 1 Tbsp. chopped tomatoes + a little extra for garnish

- 2 eggs, beaten

- 1 tsp Italian seasoning

- 1 tsp fresh Parmesan cheese

Place the egg in the pan, after you have beaten them. Once the egg starts to cook add the vegetables.

7. Walnut Pancakes

Adding walnuts to pancakes will help you boost your skin health due to the omega-3 fatty acids, according to Dr. Drayer.

Ingredients:

- 1 cup quick cooking oats
- 3 Tbsp. chopped walnuts
- ½ cup whole grain pastry flour
- 1 ½ tsp baking powder
- 1 tsp ground cinnamon
- 3 egg whites
- 1 tsp pure vanilla
- 1 scoop vanilla whey protein powder
- ½ cup fat free ricotta cheese
- ¾ cup milk

Get your skillet warming, with a little cooking spray or butter. The heat should be on low. Combine the dry ingredients and mix well. Combine the wet ingredients in a separate bowl, then add them to the dry ingredients, mixing well. Let the mix sit for 2 minutes, then start making pancakes.

8. Chocolate Banana Muffins

Research shows dark chocolate has a healthy effect on your skin by offering it hydration and decreasing scaling.

Ingredients:

- 1 ½ cup walnuts
- ¾ cup semisweet dark chocolate baking chips
- 1 ½ cup flour
- 1 Tbsp. baking powder
- ½ cup brown sugar
- ½ tsp cinnamon
- ¼ cup canola oil
- ¼ cup milk
- ¼ cup Greek yogurt (plain)
- 1 egg
- 1 ripe banana, mashed
- 1 tsp vanilla

Preheat the oven to 375 degrees F. Combine the wet ingredients in one bowl and the dry ingredients in the other. Leave the banana out for now. Combine the wet ingredients into the dry, then add the banana as the last step. Put the mix into muffin tins. Cook for 20 minutes in the oven.

9. Bagel with Lox and Cream Cheese

Lox is filled with omega 3-fatty acids, which you know helps your skin.

Ingredients:

- Use fat free cream cheese
- Smoked salmon
- Cucumber, sliced
- Tomato sliced
- Leaves of lettuce
- Choice of bagel

Using a choice of bagel, spread 1 Tbsp. of cream cheese on each side of the bagel. Place 1 to 3 ounces of salmon on the bagel. Top it will lettuce, cucumber, and tomato.

10. Quick Breakfast

Whole grains are full of antioxidants, which help your complexion. Many cereals like Total also have zinc, which is an anti-inflammatory vitamin. Using cereal combined with a banana you can increase your collagen as well as your overall skin health.

Ingredients:

- 1 cup cereal (whole grain such as Total)

- 1 banana, sliced

- Milk

- 2 tsp walnuts, chopped

Simply add each element to a bowl, with enough milk to please your palette and eat.

Chapter 2: Lunches

Your body requires a mixture of various proteins, vitamins, and minerals to be healthy and fight disease. For lunches you want to make certain you are eating a high amount of protein, fewer carbohydrates, and plenty of fruits and vegetables. The recipe suggestions in this section all focus on the main meal, but remember you can always add as many vegetables as you want not only to increase your food intake, but also to ensure your skin continues to glow.

1. Shrimp with Grapefruit

Antioxidant grapefruit again makes an appearance to help your skin glow.

Ingredients:

- 1 red grapefruit
- 1 teaspoon Dijon mustard
- ½ teaspoon Himalayan Pink Salt
- ¼ teaspoon black pepper
- 2 tablespoons olive oil
- 1 large head shredded romaine lettuce or spring mix
- 1 avocado, peeled, pitted and chopped
- 1 pound peeled, deveined and cooked large shrimp

Over a large bowl section, the grapefruit allowing juices to drip into bowl. Squeeze the grapefruit rind over the large bowl to gather all the juice. Put the sections in a smaller bowl. Whisk the mustard, salt and pepper into the large bowl with juice. Whisk in oil. Add the lettuce, avocado, shrimp and grapefruit. Toss the ingredients to coat with the juices. Serves 4

2. Tuna with White Bean Salad

Vitamin rich tomatoes are the key to good skin care in this delicious recipe.

Ingredients:

- 1/3 cup tomato juice

- 3 tablespoons lemon juice

- 2 tablespoons olive oil

- 1 tablespoon fresh basil, chopped or 1 teaspoon dried

- ¼ teaspoon salt

- 1 6-ounce can tuna, drained

- 1 can 15 ounces' white beans, drained and rinsed

- 1 medium cucumber, peeled, seeded and chopped

- ¼ cup pitted Kalamata olives, chopped

- 6 cups of mixed salad greens

In a small bowl, whisk together the first five ingredients. In a medium bowl, toss the next four ingredients with one tablespoon of vinaigrette. Divide the greens among four plates. Top with a quarter of the tuna mixture and drizzle with dressing.

3. Sweet Potato Soup

With more than 30 antioxidant compounds in ginger this sweet potato soup recipe is not only full of flavor but skin benefits as well. It removes toxins, prevents damage caused by free radicals and helps with stimulate proper circulation.

Ingredients:

- 2 tablespoon olive oil
- 2 cloves garlic, minced
- 1 large onion, chopped
- 1 red bell pepper, chopped
- 1 teaspoon ground ginger
- 1 teaspoon allspice
- 4 cups low-sodium chicken or vegetable broth
- 2 large sweet potatoes, peeled and cut into 1 inch chunks
- 1 14-ounce can diced tomatoes
- ½ cup natural peanut butter or almond butter
- 1 16-ounce frozen edamame, shelled
- 5 ounces' baby spinach

Start by warming up the broth in a pan, add in the sliced sweet potatoes. Let the potatoes cook until they are partially soft and add in the rest of the ingredients. The peanut butter will help reduce the amount of broth, making the soup a little thicker.

4. Kale Salad with Pomegranate Seeds and Lemon Vinaigrette

The ingredients in this salad provide plenty of antioxidants, including vitamin K, which are both known to help your skin look younger and fight the aging process. Pomegranate seeds also contain polyphenols, which are in tea, as well, and help with healthy skin and body.

Ingredients:

- Avocado

- Kale

- Quinoa

- Pecans

- Goat Cheese

- Lemon Vinaigrette

- Pomegranate Seeds

- Romaine lettuce

- Spinach

For 1 cup of lettuce, add in as many of the vegetables as you want, use 1 Tbsp. of pecans, 1 ounce of goat cheese, and 2 Tbsp. of the lemon vinaigrette. For the seeds, simply add 1 Tbsp.

5. Lemon Herb Salmon

You have seen salmon before in a breakfast recipe. The same principle applies here for healthier skin.

Ingredients:

- 3 ounces of Salmon
- One lemon
- Ginger
- Garlic
- Celery seeds
- Oregano

Use the herbs to taste. Simply place them over the salmon and squeeze the lemon juice onto the fish. Lay sliced lemon over the salmon, bake it at 350 degrees F until it is cooked. Depending on the thickness of the salmon it may take 10 to 20 minutes.

6. Chicken Salad with Nuts

Chicken is a healthy food, not only because it is low in cholesterol, but because of its antioxidant properties. Combine it with walnuts and cranberries and you will definitely add healthy components that help your skin.

Ingredients:

- 2 Tbsp. mayo

- ½ pound chicken

- Whole grain bread

- ¼ cup cranberries

- ¼ cup walnuts

Combine the ingredients in a bowl, with the chicken, diced, then spread the chicken salad over the bread.

7. Chicken Pot Pie

Chicken pot pie allows you to get vegetables, meat, potatoes, and crust all in one. The vegetables you use can all lend a hand in keeping your skin glowing and fight aging; especially if you combine spinach, kale, or tomatoes into your pie.

Ingredients:

- Celery

- Tomatoes

- Potatoes

- Carrots

- Chicken

- Pie crust

- Chicken Gravy

This lunch will need to be made the night before. Heat the oven to 350 degrees F. Place a crust in the bottom of a pie pan. Dice your chicken and vegetables. Put them in the pie pan in a nice even layer. Layer the ingredients with the gravy, place the second crust on the top and bake for 30 minutes. If you do not like tomatoes, spinach or kale in the pie, you can have that as your side dish such as a spinach salad.

8. Broccoli Chicken Stir-fry

Stir-fry is just a way to say you have a lot of vegetables and meat to place over Ramen or Rice. What you put in a stir fry is up to you, but if you want healthy skin, then the suggestions for this recipe will definitely provide antioxidants for your skin health, plus vitamins C, E, and A. Broccoli is also known to help with skin regeneration and repair due to a property called glucoraphanin.

Ingredients:

- 1 pound of chicken

- 2 heads of broccoli

- 1 carrot

- 1 cup of seaweed

- Peppers

- Onion

- Water chestnuts

- Bamboo shoots

- If there are any vegetables such as mushrooms that you like, you can add them. The main point is to have the broccoli and chicken in the dish. You can decide to use soy sauce or another stir-fry sauce. One with ginger is a good option since ginger also has antioxidant and anti-inflammatory properties. Brown rice is best for health reasons. Simply cook the chicken, add the carrots and other hard vegetables once the chicken is cooked. Add in the sauce and the rest of the vegetables, let cook until the vegetables are cooked and serve over rice or noodles.

9. Light Lunch Dip

Sometimes you might not want a lot for lunch, but you want it to help you keep your skin healthy. An Edamame Ginger dip can be the light lunch that you want, which is filled with antioxidants and ingredients that will keep you full.

Ingredients:

- Edamame
- 1tbsp Ginger
- 2tbsp Soy Sauce
- ¼ cup water
- 1 tbsp. rice vinegar
- 1 tbsp. tahini
- 1 clove garlic

Cook the edamame until it is soft. Usually you have to buy a frozen shelled edamame, so the instructions are on the package. Puree the edamame with the rest of the ingredients, chill it, and then serve with crackers or carrots. It can also be a dip you have as a side with chicken.

10. Tofu Peanut Wrap

Tofu is considered a healthy alternative to meat. Adding peanuts with red bell pepper and snow peas, also adds antioxidants to the meal.

Ingredients:

- Whole wheat tortilla
- 2 thinly sliced ounces of tofu
- ¼ cup sliced bell pepper
- 8 sliced snow peas
- 1 tbsp. peanut sauce
- 1 tbsp. peanuts

Spread the peanut sauce on the tortilla. Place the other ingredients over the top and fold the tortilla to your preferences.

Chapter 3: Dinners

Many of these dinners are going to contain the same vegetables, chicken, fish and tofu of the lunch recipes. The difference will be in the type of recipe to ensure you have 10 different dinner options. Keep in mind that you can do a lot with the same types of ingredients, with only minor changes to make it more Asian, American, or European.

1. Chicken Fajitas

Chicken Fajitas can be made with your health in mind. Adding vegetables, light cheese, and whole grain tortilla shells to the meal will help you keep your skin healthy.

Ingredients:

- 1 lb. chicken
- 1 green bell pepper
- 1 yellow bell pepper
- 1 red bell pepper
- 1 onion
- Fresh herbs based on your taste
- Garlic
- 1 tbsp. butter
- Whole grain tortilla

Cook the chicken in a skillet with the butter, garlic, and herbs. Add the cut up vegetables, until they are the desired doneness. Put the tortilla in another skillet to warm it up for 30 seconds. Sprinkle some cheese onto the tortilla and add in the chicken mixture. Use Pico de Gallo or Salsa as a garnish to get health benefits from tomatoes.

2. Halibut with Spinach Salad

Halibut is a white fish found on the bottom of the ocean, in cooler temperatures. It is one of the best fish to eat, if you are not a fish fan. While it is not among the highest rated fish for minerals and antioxidants, it still contains omega 3-fatty acids.

Ingredients:

- 3 oz. Halibut
- 1 lemon
- 1 tbsp. butter
- Garlic
- Spinach
- Lemon vinaigrette
- Cranberries
- Walnuts

For the halibut, you can either grill or bake it. For grilling, put the halibut on tin foil. Butter both sides, squeeze lemon on both sides, and place garlic on both sides. Wrap the tin foil and cook for 10 minutes, flip the fish and cook another 5 minutes with the tin foil open. The length of time you cook the fish may vary based on the thickness of the fish. You may need to cook the fish for less time.

In a bowl, combine spinach, romaine if you wish, cranberries, walnuts, and lemon vinaigrette.

3. Homemade Stew

Stew is not only a simple meal, but also one that offers you plenty of different vegetables. The great part about stew is that it was originally made based off of what you had in the house. This means adding in anything you want and it can be called a stew. To make this recipe healthier for your skin, some additions have been added that might not be in your typical recipe.

Ingredients:

- Beef
- Lentils (your choice)
- Brown gravy
- Potatoes
- Leaks
- Carrots
- Celery
- onion
- Kale or spinach
- Tomatoes

For the stew, start it in the morning in your crockpot. Mix up brown gravy from a powder or use beef broth. Add the stew meat, vegetables, beans, and onion. Leave the tomatoes out. The tomatoes will be for later on when you are ready to eat your stew. Let the ingredients mix, cook, and become flavorful throughout the day.

When you are ready to eat, cut up the tomatoes into slices. Using a little salt and pepper to taste, cover the tomatoes. You can eat them raw or if you like you can fry them. You would get the best results out of the raw tomato.

4. Veggie Delight

Vegetables are some of the best foods anyone can eat for a healthy glow. If you are a vegetarian or just tired of meat, you can create a veggie meal.

Ingredients:

- 1 small yellow onion, chopped

- 2 tbsp. butter

- 3 garlic gloves, crushed

- 2 large Portobello mushrooms, sliced

- 2 ½ cups button, brown or cremini mushrooms, sliced

- 1 tbsp. flour

- ½ cup cooked brown lentils, follow the package instructions

- 2 ½ cups vegetable stock

- 1 cup pearl onions, peeled

- 1 pinch of pepper and salt to taste

In a skillet, add the butter, onions, garlic, and mushrooms. Cook until the mushrooms become soft and slightly browned. Add in the lentils and cook for an additional 2 minutes. Sprinkle the flour over the mixture, stir it in, and then add the vegetable stock. Simmer the mixture for 10 minutes or until the sauce becomes thick.

5. Cashew Chicken

Cashew chicken is a favourite among Asian cultures because it provides two types of protein, plus ingredients for a healthy skin and body. Cashews are particularly helpful in the antioxidant department.

- 1 lb. of chicken, sliced

- ½ cup of cashews

- ¼ cup soy sauce

- 1/8 cup peanut sauce

- Wheat noodles

- Vegetables

- Sesame oil

Start by heating up your wok or skillet to 300 degrees or low/medium heat. Pour 1 tbsp. of sesame oil into the pan or use butter if you don't have any. Cook the chicken first. Wait until it is cooked through before adding your choice of vegetables. Any green veggies, such as broccoli, seaweed, or veggies like carrots should be used. Onions and bell peppers are also filled with appropriate nutrients for skin health. Cook the veggies until they are soft. You can also add in the soy sauce and peanut sauce to help steam the veggies. Cook the noodles per package instructions. Once all is cooked, add in the cashews, mix it up and serve.

6. Homemade Spaghetti

Homemade spaghetti sauce is a great way to ensure you have the appropriate vitamins and antioxidants from the tomatoes in your meal.

Ingredients:

- 1 cup water

- A dozen whole tomatoes

- Garlic

- Oregano

- Other herbs

- Using Italian herbs, including oregano and garlic you will season your tomatoes. The choice of herbs is up to you and what you like. Many herbs, including oregano, garlic, and parsley have antioxidants. First, you will need to boil your tomatoes in the water. Using 6 of the tomatoes, boil them until they are soft. The other six tomatoes will be pureed in a blender until a paste starts to form. Add the pureed tomatoes to the tomatoes. This will thicken the sauce. Add in the herbs and let it cook until you have a nice flavor. For the spaghetti, simply choose a whole grain noodle, cook as you normally would.

7. Chicken Lettuce Wraps

Anytime you combine green vegetables like lettuce with chicken you are helping your skin. Lettuce wraps are another Asian dish, which are already known to have health benefits beyond just skin.

Ingredients:

- 1 lb. chicken, cut into strips
- 1 cup of water
- 1 package of lettuce wrap seasoning
- 1 bell pepper
- 1 carrot
- Green onions
- Romaine lettuce

In a skillet or wok, cook the chicken. You can use butter or sesame oil to ensure the chicken does not stick to the pan. Add the seasoning and water after the chicken is cooked, along with the vegetables, save the lettuce. While the chicken is cooking, clean the Romaine lettuce, lay out entire leaves, and then put the cooked chicken concoction in a bowl. Simply put a spoonful of chicken into the lettuce and eat it. If you would like, you can use a food processor to reduce the chicken in size for an easier time eating it.

8. Pork with Apricot Sauce

Apricots are very healthy for your skin; they can also make a great addition to pork. You will want to use a lean pork roast or pork chop to keep the cholesterol down.

Ingredients:

- 1 lb. pork

- ¼ cup Dijon

- ¼ cup apricot jelly or fresh apricots

- 1 onion

- ½ cup vegetable or chicken broth

In a skillet, put the vegetable broth, and onion in and place the pork into the pan. Cook one side. After you turn the pork over, dump the Dijon mustard and apricot mixture into the skillet. If you use fresh apricots, they need to be cut into chunks and the juice squeezed into the pan. Cook until the other side of the pork is nicely cooked. It takes about 20 minutes. Serve with the sauce to help keep the pork moist.

9. Chicken and Mandarin Salad

Green vegetables, orange fruits, and chicken make a nice compliment for a light dinner.

Ingredients:

- Romaine lettuce
- Spinach
- Mandarin oranges
- Apricots
- Apples
- 1 chicken breast or 2 tenderloins
- Salad toppings of choice

For this recipe it is about combining fruit, lettuce, and chicken, so you have a complete meal all in one bowl. It is up to you whether you use croutons, wontons, fried onions, or chow mien noodles in your salads. You also want to choose a low fat dressing or vinaigrette. You can also add more fruits and vegetables like peppers, broccoli, cranberries and blueberries to the salad.

10. Spaghetti Pie

Spaghetti Pie is a casserole dish you can create. It takes a little prep, sometime in the oven, and then you have a meal you can eat quickly. The tomatoes will bring the healthy skin glow you are looking for.

Ingredients:

- Whole grain spaghetti

- Tomato sauce, preferably homemade

- Light or fat free ricotta

- Hamburger

- Mozzarella

Cook the spaghetti noodles as you would normally do. Cook the hamburger, drain the oil and fat, then combine with the sauce. You don't have to heat the sauce. Instead, you will mix the ricotta into the sauce and pour it over the hot spaghetti, mix in the noodles, put mozzarella over the top and bake it. You will need to heat the oven to 350 degrees F, put the ingredients in a pie pan, and cook for 25 to 30 minutes.

Chapter 4: Snacks

Snacks can be just as healthy, whether you eat them throughout the day or at night. You definitely need to combine plenty of vegetables and fruits in your snacks to ensure you are eating healthy. Nuts, fruits, and vegetables all contain antioxidants, anti-inflammatory, and polyphenols that help your skin glow, rejuvenate, and lose its scaly appearance. The snacks in this section will contain these properties to ensure you have a healthy glow.

1. Blueberry Fruit Salad

Blueberries are one of the highest fruits when it comes to antioxidants and skin care. Creating a fruit salad around blueberries is simple, quick, and extremely healthy.

Ingredients:

- Blueberries

- Strawberries

- Bananas

- Kiwi

- Apricots

The main ingredient should be blueberries, but really all you need to do is slice the various other fruits, put them in a bowl and decide if you wish to add a little yogurt for protein.

2. Strawberries and Cream

For this recipe, you are taking healthy strawberries and adding them to Greek yogurt. Your other options are to use heavy whip, mix it in a mixing bowl, and dip your strawberries for a little dessert. It can also be substituted with any other fruit, including oranges, apricots, pineapple, and blueberries.

3. Artichoke Dip

Artichokes are good for your health and your skin. Like many vegetables they contain powerful properties such as anti-inflammatory and antioxidants.

Ingredients:

- 1 can artichoke hearts or fresh artichoke

- 1 cup mayo

- 1 cup grated, fresh Parmesan cheese

Preheat the oven to 375 degrees F. Combine the artichoke hearts with the other two ingredients, blend in a blender to mix well and break the hearts up a little bit. Spread into a 9x13 inch pan, bake for 15 to 20 minutes and then serve warm or cold. Serve with whole grain bread or crackers.

4. Spinach Dip

Spinach is that lovely green vegetable that you should eat more of given its healthful properties, some of which have already been discussed. Like the anti-inflammatory properties of most vegetables, you also find this in spinach.

Ingredients:

- 1 cup mayo
- 1 package of leek soup mix
- 1 16-oz sour cream
- 1 4-oz can water chestnuts, finely chopped
- 10 ounces of spinach

Mix the ingredients in a bowl. Refrigerator for 6 hours and then serve. You can serve with whole grain crackers or bread.

5. Salsa and Whole Grain Chips

Making your own salsa ensures it has everything you want in it. Tomatoes, as many of the recipes have been saying are good for skin based on the antioxidants they have.

Ingredients:

- Tomatoes
- Peppers
- Onions
- Jalapenos
- Tomato juice

Dice up the tomatoes and other vegetables as small as you wish. You can leave it as a chunky salsa or even use a food processor to reduce the size of the vegetables. Use the tomato juice from the tomatoes to mix the salsa. The amount of peppers and jalapenos will determine how spicy the food is. For every tomato you use, add the same amount as the other vegetables. The chips should be a whole grain choice.

6. Yellow and Orange Fruit Salad

Fruit salads can truly be made with anything you wish. If you are looking for more of a dessert than a fruit bowl, consider the following fruits combined with cream cheese and sweetened condensed milk.

Ingredients:

- 1 8-ounce cream cheese

- ½ can sweetened condensed milk

- 1 can mandarin oranges

- 1 orange

- ½ cup pineapple

- 1 peach

- 1 banana

Any yellow and orange fruit will be rich in antioxidants and help promote skin health. You can leave out some of the fruit or add in more. Let the cream cheese reach room temperature, so you can whip it. Add the condensed milk to make a nice, slightly runny mixture and then add all the fruit.

7. Carrots, Broccoli, and Dip

While not strictly a recipe, getting a vegetable platter with carrots, broccoli, radishes, peppers, and celery can make a nice snack. You can also create your own platter from home grown vegetables. The dip should be homemade too, for better quality.

You can use spinach or artichoke dip or the following:

- 1 cup sour cream

- 1 package ranch mix or herbs you grow

Combine the ingredients, let it sit in the fridge for an hour and serve.

8. Homemade Trail Mix

Trail mix by definition is full of nuts and fruits. There is nothing better than making your own trail mix. You can even put a few dark chocolate pieces in to help with your skin care.

- ½ cup raisins

- ½ cup walnuts

- ½ cup pecans

- ½ cup cashews

- ½ cup dried fruits (choose bananas, blueberries, cranberries, or any fruits)

- ½ cup dark chocolate pieces

Take all the ingredients, put them in a bag, shake it up, and eat it whenever you feel hungry.

9. Tuna Finger Sandwiches

Tuna is one of the best fish to make into a sandwich for a snack. You can make little finger sandwiches to serve on whole grain bread when you host a party, tea, or simply when you want a snack for the whole family.

- 1 package of Tuna

- 2 tbsp mayo, light or fat free

- Whole grain bread

Cut the bread with cookie cutters, making sure to also cut the crust off. Mix the tuna and mayo, spread it on the bread and serve. You can also add pits of celery if you prefer. Another option is to top the top piece of bread with a small green, yellow, or red pepper. It gives you another boost of antioxidants.

10. Cucumber Sandwiches and Slices

The great thing about cucumber is its anti-inflammatory properties. You can put slices on your eyes, let it help with the bags you have, and then eat the cucumber that is leftover to get even more antioxidants and anti-inflammatory properties.

For the recipe:

Ingredients:

- 1 cucumber
- Cream cheese
- Whole grain bread
- Salt and pepper

To make the sandwiches, use a cookie cutter to get little finger sandwich sizes and cut the crust off. Then spread a thin layer of cream cheese on the bread. This will hold the cucumber in place. You can add salt and pepper to enhance the taste or a little paprika. If you do not want to make a sandwich, simply salt and pepper the cucumber and eat the slices.

Chapter 5: Smoothies

Smoothies are a great way to replace a meal or snack. The right smoothie might have 300 calories with plenty of green vegetables to ensure your healthy skin will continue as you age. The smoothies in this chapter will examine various options from green smoothies to super food smoothies that will definitely contain the antioxidants, anti-inflammatory, and collagen you need to look great.

1. A Very Green Smoothie

If you want to be healthy; especially, to increase the health of your skin, then consider this green smoothie. It doesn't have a great taste, but it will rejuvenate your skin.

Ingredients:

- 1 cup spinach
- 1 small cucumber
- ½ avocado
- 1 leaf from collard greens
- 1 ½ cup water
- 1 leaf from black kale
- ¼ granny smith apple
- 2 lemons

Mix it all in a blender. Add almond or coconut milk to reduce the acidity.

2. Aloe and Apple Delight

Aloe has always been known as the healing plant. Topically, it can help heal cuts faster, as well as prevent scars. Drinking it in a smoothie also helps some of the properties reach your internal cells, particularly to help regenerate new skin cells.

Ingredients:

- 4 collard leaves

- 2 large spears of Aloe, fresh from a plant

- 1-inch fresh ginger, peeled

- 1 banana

- 1 granny smith apple

- 1 ¾ cup ice

- 1 ½ cup blueberries, fresh

Mix everything in the blender. Serve or keep for 24 hours. Adding honey for a little sweetener can also help your skin.

3. Seaweed Asian Smoothie

Seaweed like nori, wakame, and arame are known to contain antioxidants and nutrients that are helpful for the skin as well as your heart. This smoothie can help prevent certain diseases as it lowers cholesterol and adds anti-inflammatory properties to your body.

Ingredients:

- 2 handfuls of arugula
- 1 handful of spinach
- ¼ cup seaweed
- 2 cups pineapple, fresh
- 2 bananas, fresh
- 1 apple
- 3 cups ice
- 2 cups blueberries, fresh

Mix everything in a blender. It makes 3 servings and can be kept for 24 hours.

4. Asian Vegetable Smoothie with Fruit

Bok choy is known for its antioxidants and healthy properties to ensure heart health and prevention of certain diseases. In a smoothie with vegetables and fruits it can also help with your skin.

Ingredients:

- 1 cup Chinese celery
- 8 cups Bok choy, chopped
- 1 cup bean sprouts
- 4 tangelos
- 4 cups mixed berries, fresh
- 2 bananas, fresh

Mix it all in a blender with 2 ¼ cups ice. It will serve 6 people or can be kept for 24 hours.

5. Fruit and Cabbage Smoothie

This smoothie combines the properties of cabbage with fruit to help enhance your skin.

Ingredients:

- 2 cups berries or other fruit
- 1 banana
- ½ green cabbage
- 1 granny smith apple
- 1 ¾ cups ice
- ¼ cup raw agave

Put everything in the blender and mix until smooth.

6. Green Tea Fruit Smoothie

Green tea or any tea has antioxidants and anti-inflammatory properties. Mixing a little green tea infused water in with yellow, orange, or green fruits will ensure a great smoothie for your skin.

Ingredients:

- Brew 1 tsp. green tea and let it cool

- Grab whatever fruits you love in the colour categories named

- Coconut milk

Put ½ a cup of green tea in a blender, add half a dozen ice cubes, and as much fruit choices as you want. Add a tablespoon of coconut milk for the antioxidant properties and protein. Blend well. Use the left over green tea added to flour for a facial mask. You have two skin remedies in one.

7. Tofu and Vegetable Smoothie

You might need to be a hard core vegetarian for this smoothie or like tofu a lot. The vegetables help bring important properties into your body for better skin health. Tofu is great for its protein component.

- 1-ounce tofu

- Spinach and any other green vegetable you like

- Yogurt or coconut milk

In a blender put some ice, the vegetables you like, the tofu, and add enough milk to blend the concoction smooth.

8. Pomegranate, Apple, and Mango Smoothie

All three fruits have the same properties as most fruit, meaning antioxidants, vitamin C and D, which all help healthy skin promotion.

Ingredients:

- 1 fruit (apple, mango, and pomegranate)

- Yogurt, low fat milk or coconut milk

- Ice

De-seed the fruits, put them in a blender, add a cup of milk or yogurt and half a dozen ice cubes. Blend until smooth.

9. Vanilla Kefir and Orange Fruit Smoothie

Vanilla kefir is a drinkable yogurt to add to your smoothie. It has calcium and probiotics to help keep your immune system in check. Add in orange for the vitamin C and D, plus antioxidants for your skin.

Ingredients:

- 2 oranges
- 1 cup vanilla kefir

Blend until smooth in a blender and drink.

10. Whey Protein Vegetable Smoothie

Whey protein for some does not have that great a taste, but it offers you protein in a smoothie, so you can quickly have a well-balanced meal as you move about during your day. The vegetables will enhance your skin health.

Ingredients:

- 1 tbsp. whey protein
- Spinach
- Broccoli
- Kale
- Ice
- ½ cup yogurt

Combine all the ingredients into a blender, mix well, and serve.

Conclusion

Finally...

Thank you again for purchasing my book!

I hope this book was able to improve your skin, help with your food choices and ultimately make you healthier. Once you make changes to your diet, don't expect an overnight transformation. It takes around six weeks for new skin to emerge up to the surface so the visible benefits from dietary changes will take just as long. Here are two great tips to speeding up the process to getting radiant skin.

Water

Your body is composed of about 60% water and is excellent for keeping skin looking at its best:

- Water aids digestion, absorption, circulation, creation of saliva, transportation of nutrients, and maintenance of body temperature.
- Your skin contains plenty of water and functions as a protective barrier to avert excess fluid loss.
- Dehydration makes your skin look more dry and wrinkled.
- When you are getting enough fluids, urine flows freely, is light in color and free of odor.
- When your body is not getting sufficient fluids, urine concentration, color and odor increases because the kidneys trap extra fluid for bodily functions.

The Institute of Medicine concluded that an adequate intake for men is roughly about 13 cups or 3 liters of total beverages a day. The ideal intake for women is about 9 cups 2.2 liters of total beverages a day. This should predominantly be water as this is the purest liquid and is perfect for keeping skin truly glowing.

Exercise

Exercise is a fantastic way to help skin look amazing along with a great diet and adequate water. So I certainly recommend doing something each day to get the heart going and the benefits range from:

- Reduce cellulite
- Lift your libido
- Reverse the ageing process
- Sleep better
- Combat spots
- Enjoy luscious locks

The next step is read over the ingredients, snacks and ingredients of the meals included here so when you go to your local shops you can select the best food for your skin.

Finally, if you enjoyed this book, please take the time to share your thoughts and post a review on Amazon. It'd be greatly appreciated!

Thank you and good luck!

Check out the handy books to help with your health and skin nutrition:

Amazing Home Remedies for Acne, Symptoms Causes and Remedies For Acne

How to Build Muscle with Vegetarian Meals: 21 Protein-Packed Recipes

How To Build The Female Fitness Model Body: Building A Female Fitness Model Physique, Female Fitness Model Workout and Training Regime

The Woman's Health Book: 6 Week 16:8 Fasting Diet and Training, Sexier Leaner Healthier You!

www.ingramcontent.com/pod-product-compliance
Lightning Source LLC
Chambersburg PA
CBHW071249280526
45788CB00004B/1641